Table of Contents

Introduction

5

Pancreatitis is an inflammation of the pancreas that occurs when pancreatic enzyme secretions build up and begin to digest the organ itself. It can occur as acute, painful attacks lasting a matter of days, or it may be a chronic, condition that progresses over a period of years.

Management of acute pancreatitis in the early stages is supportive. Intravenous fluid replacement has an important role but the type and rate of administration of the fluid is unclear. The role of antibiotics in preventing infection is highly debated. It is recognised that patients who develop infected pancreatic necrosis should

5

undergo a form of drainage or necrosectomy to treat this but the type of intervention for each patient is unclear. Indications for referral to a specialist pancreatic centre are variable and require clarification.

Chronic pancreatitis causes a significant reduction in pancreatic function and a majority of people have reduced exocrine (digestive) function and reduced endocrine function (causing diabetes). They may need expert dietary advice and medication.

Chronic pancreatitis can also give rise to specific complications including painful inflammatory mass and obstructed pancreatic duct, biliary or duodenal obstruction and haemorrhage.

People with pancreatitis are at long-term risk of nutritional problems and diabetes, and also have an increased risk of pancreatic cancer, which is even higher in people with hereditary pancreatitis. It is necessary to identify those who need to be followed up and what tests are required.

Pancreatitis is a serious and complex condition. It causes immense suffering, can have a severe effect on quality of life and may result in reduced life expectancy. In the past, there has been lack of knowledge on how to manage pancreatitis and this has resulted in clinicians avoiding those with the disease and conflicting advice being offered. With this guideline it is hoped that sound advice will be provided to enable people with pancreatitis to receive appropriate care to improve the outcomes from this difficult condition.

The Pancreas and Its Functions

The pancreas is an organ located in the abdomen. It plays an essential role in converting the food we eat into fuel for the body's cells. The pancreas has two main functions: an exocrine function that helps in digestion and an endocrine function that regulates blood sugar.

Functions of the Pancreas

A healthy pancreas produces the correct chemicals in the proper quantities, at the right times, to digest the foods we eat.

Exocrine Function:

The pancreas contains exocrine glands that produce enzymes important to digestion. These enzymes include trypsin and chymotrypsin to digest proteins; amylase for the digestion of carbohydrates; and lipase to break down fats. When food enters the stomach, these pancreatic juices are released into a system of ducts that culminate in the main pancreatic duct. The pancreatic duct joins the common bile duct to form the ampulla of Vater which is located at the first portion of the small intestine, called the duodenum. The common bile duct originates in the liver and the gallbladder and produces another important digestive juice called bile. The pancreatic juices and bile that are released into the duodenum, help the body to digest fats, carbohydrates, and proteins.

Endocrine Function:

The endocrine component of the pancreas consists of islet cells (islets of Langerhans) that create and release important hormones directly into the bloodstream. Two of the main pancreatic hormones are insulin, which acts to lower blood sugar, and glucagon, which acts to raise blood sugar. Maintaining proper blood sugar levels is crucial to the functioning of key organs including the brain, liver, and kidneys.

Location of the Pancreas

The pancreas is located behind the stomach in the upper left abdomen. It is surrounded by other organs including the small intestine, liver, and spleen. It is spongy, about six to ten inches long, and is shaped like a flat pear or a fish extended horizontally across the abdomen.

The wide part, called the head of the pancreas, is positioned toward the center of the abdomen. The head of the pancreas is located at the juncture where the stomach meets the first part of the small intestine. This is where the stomach empties partially digested food into the intestine, and the pancreas releases digestive enzymes into these contents.

The central section of the pancreas is called the neck or body.

The thin end is called the tail and extends to the left side.

Almost all of the pancreas (95%) consists of exocrine tissue that produces pancreatic enzymes for digestion. The remaining tissue consists of endocrine cells called islets of Langerhans. These clusters of cells look like grapes and produce hormones that regulate blood sugar and regulate pancreatic secretions.

Diseases of the Pancreas

Disorders affecting the pancreas include pancreatitis, precancerous conditions such as PanIN and IPMN, and pancreatic cancer. Each disorder may exhibit different symptoms and requires different treatments.

Precursors to Pancreatic Cancer

The exact cause of pancreatic cancer is still unknown, but there are known risk factors that increase the risk of developing the disease. Cigarette smoking, a family history of pancreatic cancer or hereditary cancer syndromes, and chronic pancreatitis are some of these factors. In addition, certain pancreatic lesions such as Intraductal Papillary Mucinous Neoplasms (IPMNs) and Pancreatic Intraepithelial Neoplasia (PanIN) are considered precursors to pancreatic cancer.

Types of Pancreatitis

There are different types of Pancreatitis:

1. Acute Pancreatitis

2. Chronic Pancreatitis

3. Autoimmune Pancreatitis

4. Viral Pancreatitis

5. Parasitic Pancreatitis

Acute Pancreatitis

Acute pancreatitis refers to pancreatitis that develops suddenly, most often as a result of gallstones or alcohol ingestion. Reaction to certain medications, trauma, and infectious causes can also lead to acute pancreatitis. Acute pancreatitis can be life threatening, but most patients recover completely.

Chronic Pancreatitis

Chronic pancreatitis refers to ongoing disease in which the pancreas continues to sustain damage and lose function over time. The majority of cases of chronic pancreatitis result from ongoing alcohol abuse, but some cases are hereditary or due to diseases such as cystic fibrosis.

Autoimmune Pancreatitis

In approximately 5-6% of patients with chronic pancreatitis, the disease is caused by autoimmune inflammation (in which the immune system attacks the pancreas). Symptoms may be mild, but patients with autoimmune pancreatitits (AIP) tend to show elevated levels of immunoglobulin G4 (IgG4) and a high rate of pancreatic stone formation. Other indicators of autoimmune pancreatitis include narrowing of the main pancreatic duct, scarring of the pancreatic tissue, and infiltration with inflammatory cells. AIP can occur by itself or in association with other autoimmune diseases such as primary sclerosing cholangitis (PSC), primary biliary cirrhosis, retroperitoneal fibrosis, rheumatoid arthritis, sarcoidosis, and Sjögren's syndrome.

Viral Pancreatitis

In rare cases, pancreatitis may be caused by viral infections such as mumps, coxsackie B, mycoplasma pneumonia, and campylobacter.

Parasitic Pancreatitis

A more common problem in developing countries than in the U.S., intestinal parasites can lead to acute pancreatitis and other pancreatic diseases.

Symptoms of Acute Pancreatitis

- Severe, steady pain in the upper-middle part of the abdomen, often radiating into the back

- Jaundice

- Low-grade fever

- Nausea or vomiting

- Lowered blood pressure

- Clammy skin

- Unusual abdominal hardness or mass that can be felt

- Abdominal bloating and tenderness

- Bruising (ecchymosis) in the flanks and midsection

- The tissue of the pancreas may become necrotic (tissue death)

- Pancreatic abscess

- Pancreatic pseudocyst, which is an abnormal deposit of tissue, fluid and debris that can result after episodes of acute pancreatitis, typically 1 to 4 weeks after onset

Symptoms of Chronic Pancreatitis

Symptoms may develop over a period of time without the sudden dramatic occurrence of an acute attack. However, those with undiagnosed chronic pancreatitis may develop acute episodes. In chronic pancreatitis, there is a decrease in the secretion of enzymes needed for digestion and absorption of dietary fats. Fat digestion is impaired, resulting in fatty stools. This is called exocrine insufficiency. Recurrent abdominal pain may be accompanied by nausea and weight loss. Diagnostic scans may find stones or areas of calcified tissue within the pancreas.

Symptoms of chronic pancreatitis include:

- Abdominal and/or back pain

- Weight loss

- Nausea and vomiting

- Onset of diabetes mellitus

- Pale colored, oily stools

Causes of Pancreatitis Generally

In more than half of patients, chronic pancreatitis is caused by long-term abuse of alcohol, which leads to damage and scarring of the pancreas. Other people may develop chronic pancreatitis as a result of hereditary causes and other causes, including:

- Gallstones

- Structural problems of the pancreatic and bile ducts

- Some medications like estrogen supplements and some diuretics

- Severe viral or bacterial infection

Causes of Acute Pancreatitis

Acute pancreatitis is most commonly caused by gallstones or heavy alcohol consumption. Other causes may include use of certain medications (such as immunosuppressants, estrogens, thiazide diuretics, and azathioprine), lipid (triglyceride) disorders, infections, surgery, or trauma to the abdomen from an accident or injury. Acute pancreatitis is considered idiopathic (cause is unknown) in 10 to 15% of patients.

Causes of Chronic Pancreatitis

In more than half of patients, chronic pancreatitis is caused by long-term abuse of alcohol, which leads to damage and scarring of the pancreas. Other people may develop chronic pancreatitis as a result of hereditary causes, gallstones (which block the pancreatic duct outlet), autoimmune disease such as lupus, or high triglyceride levels. The cause of chronic pancreatitis cannot be identified in about 25 -30% of patients. Evidence suggests that some cases of unidentified chronic pancreatitis may be associated with atypical mutations of cystic fibrosis genes.

Diagnosing Pancreatitis

Pancreatitis may be suspected if a patient experiences symptoms and has risk factors such as heavy alcohol use or gallstones. A number of tests and procedures may be performed to determine how well the pancreas is functioning.

Laboratory Tests

Blood testing may be done to measure digestive enzymes. Elevated levels of amylase and lipase can suggest acute pancreatitis.

Blood testing may also be used to test the patient's blood glucose levels, to determine whether the insulin-producing cells of the pancreas are functioning normally or not.

Stool testing to measure the level of elastase, an enzyme produced by the pancreas that helps to digest proteins.

Radiology

CT scan to check for complications such as infection or fluid around the pancreas;

Abdominal ultrasound to check for gallstones.

Magnetic Resonance Cholangiopancreatography: a form of MRI that is used to visualize the bile ducts and the pancreatic duct.

Diagnostic Procedures

Endoscopic Retrograde Cholangiopancreatography (ERCP):

placement of a tube down the throat, into the stomach, and into the small intestine. Using contrast dye and x-ray, ERCP allows visualization of the pancreatic and bile ducts. If gallstones are blocking the bile duct, they can be removed during ERCP.

Endoscopic Ultrasound:

Placement of a lighted scope down the throat and into the stomach to visualize the pancreas and abdominal organs. Endoscopic ultrasound may reveal gallstones and can be helpful in diagnosing severe pancreatitis (while an invasive test such as ERCP might make the condition worse). A biopsy (removal of small portion of tissue) may be performed during endoscopic ultrasound.

Pancreatitis Treatments

Treatment for acute pancreatitis may include nutritional support with feeding tubes or intravenous (IV) nutrition, antibiotics, and pain medications. Surgery is sometimes needed to treat complications. Treatment for chronic pancreatitis may involve IV fluids; pain medication; a low-fat, nutritious diet; and enzyme supplements. Surgery may be necessary to remove part or all of the pancreas.

IV fluids, Enteral Nutrition, TPN

To allow the pancreas to recover and to prevent damage and irritation, patients with pancreatitis may need to temporarily receive intravenous fluids for hydration. If you are unable to eat for more than 5-7 days, or if you are malnourished, you may begin enteral nutrition via a small tube placed through the nose. This will deliver nutrition formula to your stomach or small intestines. Sometimes enteral nutrition is contraindicated or not tolerated. Under these circumstances, parenteral (intravenous) nutrition is indicated, and is better than no nutrition.

Stents

The bile duct is a small tube that carries bile, which is produced in the liver, from the liver and gall-bladder to the small intestine. The pancreatic ducts are small tubes that carry pancreatic juices to the small intestine. These fluids help to break down food, and the two ducts usually join before emptying into the small intestine. If the ducts are narrowed or blocked due to gallstones, a tumor, infection, scarring, pseudocysts, or other trauma or illness, the fluids can build up and cause pancreatitis.

It may be necessary to open the blocked bile or pancreatic duct using a stent, which is a small plastic or metal tube placed within the duct to keep it open.

ERCP

Endoscopic retrograde cholangiopancreatography (ERCP) is a procedure that combines upper gastrointestinal (GI) endoscopy and x rays to diagnose and treat pancreatitis and other problems of the pancreatic ducts. ERCP may be performed if a person's bile or pancreatic ducts are suspected of being narrowed or blocked due to pancreatitis or other causes.

During ERCP, a flexible, lighted endoscope is inserted into the esophagus, through the stomach, and into the duodenum (the first part of the small intestine). Contrast dye is injected into the ducts, and x-ray video (fluoroscopy) allows physicians to see any areas of narrowed or blocked flow from the bile duct or pancreatic ducts. If a problem is found, the physicians can then insert special tools through the endoscope to open blocked ducts, break up or remove gallstones, remove tumors in the ducts, or insert stents to restore the flow of pancreatic or bile fluid. A biopsy may also be taken through the endoscope, in order to evaluate cells for infection or cancer.

If gallstones are the cause of pancreatitis, they may be removed during ERCP, to be followed by removal of the gallbladder (called cholecystectomy).

Enzyme Supplementation

The pancreas is normally stimulated to release pancreatic enzymes when there is undigested food in the intestine. These enzymes join with bile and begin breaking down food in the small intestine.

Enzyme supplements begin predigesting food while it is in the stomach, helping to reduce stimulation of the pancreas caused by food intake.

If a patient has digestive enzyme deficiency, enzyme supplements help food to be better absorbed, which improves nutritional intake. Avoiding stimulation of the pancreas also helps to reduce pain associated with pancreatitis.

Pain Management

The Pancreas Management Centers work to find the optimal pain management regimen that enables each patient to remain active and at home rather than in the hospital or unable to maintain normal levels of activity.

Many patients take a regimen of more than one kind of medication. Oral medications include narcotics such as Percocet and oxycodone, and these may be used in conjunction with non-narcotic medicines such as muscle relaxants and antidepressants. Oral methadone is a very good medication for managing chronic pain.

Once an oral regimen is established, acute flare-ups can be managed by temporarily adding medications. If oral medicines can't be tolerated, patients may need to be admitted to the hospital for intravenous medications. Nerve blocks may be used to manage pain for several months at a time: nerve blocks entail the insertion of a needle through the skin in the back to block the signals of the main nerves going to the pancreas. This procedure can also be done endoscopically, in which the bundle of nerves to the pancreas is injected with long-acting pain medication that lasts several months. This is performed using an endoscope through the stomach. Nerve blocks destroy the nerves, but in time they grow back so patients need repeated treatments.

Another approach to managing pain is the use of implantable pain pumps in the spine. Most implantable pumps deliver constant low doses to keep pain manageable, and they may be used in conjunction with oral medications.

Importance of Taking Pain Medications

Some patients express concern about not wanting to become addicted to pain medications. It is important to understand that severe ongoing pain needs to be addressed so that patients can maintain active lives, and a true need for pain medication does not constitute a psychological addiction. Some patients must always use medications, because chronic pancreatitis does not go away and the pain needs to be managed in order for them to function. When chronic pancreatitis is caused by microscopic inflammation of the pancreas, management of ongoing pain does not constitute a social addiction, but rather it is a needed therapy like taking blood pressure medication. Our team tries to use constellations of different medications in order to keep narcotic dosages as low as possible.

Surgery

Depending on the cause of pancreatitis, the patient's anatomy, level of pain, and other factors, surgery may be an appropriate treatment.

If gallstones are the cause of pancreatitis, surgery to remove the gallstones and possibly the gallbladder may be required. Surgery may be needed to drain pseudocysts, or accumulations of fluid and tissue in the pancreatic area.

Removal of the entire pancreas (total pancreatectomy) may be performed in order to reduce or eliminate intractable pain associated with chronic pancreatitis. Total Pancreatectomy relieves pain in 90% of cases, but causes patients to become diabetic.

To improve the lives of patients who undergo pancreatectomy, the Pancreas Center now offers autologous islet cell transplantation, an innovative process of extracting the patient's own insulin-producing cells and then reinjecting them into the liver after removal of the pancreas. By reinfusing the pancreatic islet cells, this procedure may allow patients to retain some of their insulin-producing function, thereby preventing the difficult-to-treat form of diabetes known as brittle diabetes.

Pancreatitis Diet

Nutrition is a vitally important part of treatment for patients with pancreatitis. The primary goals of nutritional management for chronic pancreatitis are:

- Prevent malnutrition and nutritional deficiencies

- Maintain normal blood sugar levels (avoid both hypoglycemia and hyperglycemia)

- Prevent or optimally manage diabetes, kidney problems, and other conditions associated with chronic pancreatitis

- Avoid causing an acute episode of pancreatitis

To best achieve those goals, it is important for pancreatitis patients to eat high protein, nutrient-dense diets that include fruits, vegetables, whole grains, low fat dairy, and other lean protein sources. Abstinence from alcohol and greasy or fried foods is important in helping to prevent malnutrition and pain.

Nutritional assessments and dietary modifications are made on an individual basis because each patient's condition is unique and requires an individualized plan.

Pancreatitis Program offers nutritional and gastrointestinal support for those with pancreatitis.

Vitamins & Minerals

Patients with chronic pancreatitis are at high risk for malnutrition due to malabsorption and depletion of nutrients as well as due to increased metabolic activity. Malnutrition can be further affected by ongoing alcohol abuse and pain after eating. Vitamin deficiency from malabsorption can cause osteoporosis, digestive problems, abdominal pain, and other symptoms.

Therefore, patients with chronic pancreatitis must be tested regularly for nutritional deficiencies. Vitamin therapies should be based on these annual blood tests. In general, multivitamins, calcium, iron, folate, vitamin E, vitamin A, vitamin D, and vitamin B12 may be supplemented, depending on the results of blood work.

If you have malnutrition, you may benefit from working with our Registered Dietitian who can guide you towards a personalized diet plan.

Risk of diabetes in chronic pancreatitis

Chronic pancreatitis also causes the pancreas to gradually lose its ability to function properly, and endocrine function will eventually be lost. This puts patients at risk for type 1 diabetes. Patients should therefore avoid refined sugars and simple carbohydrates.

Enzyme Supplementation

If pancreatic enzymes are prescribed, it is important to take them regularly in order to prevent flare-ups.

The healthy pancreas is stimulated to release pancreatic enzymes when undigested food reaches the small intestine. These enzymes join with bile and begin breaking down food in the small intestine.

Since your pancreas is not working optimally, you may not be getting the pancreatic enzymes you need to digest your food properly. Taking enzymes can help to digest your food, thus improving any signs or symptoms of steatorrhea (excess fat in the stool, or fat malabsorption). In turn this will improve your ability to eat better, lowering your risk for malnutrition.

What to Avoid

Alcohol

If pancreatitis was caused by alcohol use, you should abstain from alcohol. If other causes of acute pancreatitis have been addressed and resolved (such as via gallbladder removal) and the pancreas returned to normal, you should be able to lead a normal life, but alcohol should still be taken only in moderation (maximum of 1 serving/day). In chronic pancreatitis, there is ongoing inflammation and malabsorption — patients gradually lose digestive function and eventually lose insulin function — so regular use of alcohol is unwise.

Smoking

People with pancreatitis should avoid smoking, as it increases the risk for pancreatic cancer.

What to Eat if You Have Pancreatitis

To get your pancreas healthy, focus on foods that are rich in protein, low in animal fats, and contain antioxidants. Try lean meats, beans and lentils, clear soups, and dairy alternatives (such as flax milk and almond milk). Your pancreas won't have to work as hard to process these.

Research suggests that some people with pancreatitis can tolerate up to 30 to 40% of calories from fat when it's from whole-food plant sources or medium-chain triglycerides (MCTs). Others do better with much lower fat intake, such as 50 grams or less per day.

1. Spinach

2. Blueberries

3. cherries, and

4. whole grains can work to protect your digestion and fight the free radicals that damage your organs.

Note: If you're craving something sweet, reach for fruit instead of added sugars since those with pancreatitis are at high risk for diabetes.

Also consider the following:

1. cherry tomatoes

2. cucumbers and hummus and

3. fruit as your go-to snacks. Your pancreas will thank you.

What Not To Eat If You Have Pancreatitis

Foods to limit include:

- red meat

- organ meats

- fried foods

- fries and potato chips

- mayonnaise

- margarine and butter

- full-fat dairy

- pastries and desserts with added sugars

- beverages with added sugars

If you're trying to combat pancreatitis, avoid trans-fatty acids in your diet.

Fried or heavily processed foods, like french fries and fast-food hamburgers, are some of the worst offenders. Organ meats, full-fat dairy, potato chips, and mayonnaise also top the list of foods to limit.

Cooked or deep-fried foods might trigger a flare-up of pancreatitis. You'll also want to cut back on the refined flour found in cakes, pastries, and cookies. These foods can tax the digestive system

by causing your insulin levels to spike.